I0711353

A Nurse's Essential Planner for Care, Compassion

Streamline Your Patient Care with Comprehensive Scheduling, Assessment, and Resource Management

Kitchen Mage

Copyright © [2024] by [Kitchen Mage]. All rights reserved. No part of this index may be reproduced, distributed, or transmitted in any form or by any means, including photocopying, recording, or other electronic or mechanical methods, without the prior written permission of the publisher, except in the case of brief quotations embodied in critical reviews and certain other noncommercial uses permitted by copyright law.

The target audiences

1. Registered Nurses (RNs) working in hospitals
2. Nurse Practitioners (NPs) in primary care settings
3. Nurse Managers overseeing nursing staff
4. Nursing Students learning about patient care organization
5. Home Health Nurses managing multiple patient schedules
6. Hospice Nurses providing end-of-life care
7. School Nurses coordinating care for students
8. Nurse Educators teaching organizational skills to students
9. Community Health Nurses serving diverse populations
10. Specialty Nurses in fields such as oncology, cardiology, or pediatrics.
11. Case Managers coordinating care for patients across different healthcare settings
12. Nurse Administrators overseeing healthcare facilities and programs

13. Nurse Entrepreneurs developing innovative care coordination solutions
14. Nurse Consultants providing expertise in care planning and organization
15. Nurse Researchers studying the effectiveness of care coordination strategies
16. Public Health Nurses focusing on population-level health promotion and disease prevention
17. Nurse Leaders Advocating for Improvements in Patient Care Processes
18. Nurse Coaches supporting other nurses in developing effective care plans
19. Nursing Assistants assisting with patient care and scheduling tasks
20. Nurse Volunteers providing services in underserved communities.

Table of Contents

Chapter 2: Scheduling Mastery

- Strategies for managing busy nursing schedules effectively
- Utilizing time management techniques to prioritize tasks and appointments
- Tips for avoiding burnout and maintaining work-life balance

Chapter 3: Assessment and Documentation

- Guidance on thorough and accurate patient assessment
- Best practices for documenting patient information and care plans
- Using technology to enhance assessment and documentation processes

Chapter 4: Care Coordination Essentials

- Techniques for collaborating with interdisciplinary teams
- Effective communication strategies with patients, families, and colleagues
- Resources for navigating complex healthcare systems and referrals

Chapter 5: Resource Management

- Maximizing resources to optimize patient care outcomes
- Budgeting tips for managing healthcare resources efficiently
- Incorporating evidence-based practices and guidelines into care planning

Chapter 6: Self-Care and Professional Development

- Importance of self-care for nurses' physical, emotional, and mental well-being
- Strategies for managing stress and preventing compassion fatigue
- Opportunities for professional growth and continuing education

Chapter 7: Ethical Considerations in Care Planning

- Discussion on ethical dilemmas nurses may encounter in care planning and coordination
- Strategies for addressing ethical issues while upholding patient autonomy and dignity
- Case studies illustrating ethical decision-making in nursing practice

Chapter 8: Cultural Competence and Diversity in Patient Care

- Importance of cultural competence in providing holistic and respectful care
- Tips for navigating cultural differences and language barriers in care planning
- Promoting diversity and inclusion in healthcare settings

Chapter 9: Technology Integration for Enhanced Care Coordination

- Overview of digital tools and software designed to streamline care coordination
- Tips for selecting and implementing technology solutions that meet nurses' needs
- Ethical considerations and privacy concerns related to electronic health records and Telehealth

Chapter 10: Emergency Preparedness and Crisis Management

- Strategies for developing emergency response plans and protocols
- Role of nurses in disaster preparedness and mitigation efforts
- Case studies highlighting effective crisis management in healthcare settings

Chapter 11: Quality Improvement and Patient Safety

- Importance of quality improvement initiatives in enhancing patient outcomes
- Techniques for monitoring and evaluating the effectiveness of care plans
- Implementing evidence-based practices to improve patient safety and satisfaction

Chapter 12: Leadership and Advocacy in Nursing

- Opportunities for nurses to take on leadership roles in care planning and coordination
- Advocacy strategies for promoting policy changes and improving healthcare systems
- Inspiring stories of nurse leaders making a difference in their communities

Chapter 13: Innovations in Nursing Practice

- Exploration of innovative approaches to care planning and coordination
- Examples of nurse-led initiatives and projects driving positive change in healthcare
- Tips for embracing creativity and embracing new ideas in nursing practice

Chapter 14: Future Trends and Challenges in Nursing

- Discussion on emerging trends and challenges shaping the future of nursing practice
- Opportunities for nurses to adapt and thrive in an evolving healthcare landscape
- Recommendations for staying informed and prepared for future developments

Chapter 15: Reflection and Goal Setting

- Encouragement for nurses to reflect on their practice and personal growth
- Tools and exercises for setting short-term and long-term goals in care planning and coordination
- Strategies for celebrating achievements and maintaining motivation in nursing practice.

Conclusion

- Recap of key concepts and tools provided in the planner
- Encouragement for nurses to prioritize care, compassion, and coordination in their practice
- Invitation to share feedback and success stories using the planner

Appendix: Additional Resources

- Templates for care plans, assessment forms, and scheduling tools
- Recommended readings, websites, and organizations for further learning and support

Index

- A comprehensive index for easy reference to specific topics and tools throughout the book.

Introduction

In the dynamic landscape of healthcare, effective care planning and coordination stand as fundamental pillars of nursing practice. As frontline caregivers, nurses play a pivotal role in ensuring the delivery of safe, comprehensive, and patient-centered care. Central to this responsibility is the ability to navigate intricate patient needs, manage resources efficiently, and foster seamless collaboration within interdisciplinary teams.

This introduction serves as a compass, guiding nurses toward a deeper understanding of the critical importance of meticulous care planning and coordination in their daily practice. By laying a solid foundation in these essential skills, nurses can enhance patient outcomes, optimize resource utilization, and cultivate a culture of excellence in healthcare delivery.

Within the pages of this planner lies a comprehensive toolkit meticulously crafted to empower nurses in their mission to provide exemplary care. Designed with the intricacies of nursing practice in mind, this planner serves as a trusted companion, offering practical guidance, customizable templates, and insightful strategies tailored to the diverse needs of healthcare professionals.

Through the systematic integration of scheduling mastery, assessment and documentation proficiency, care coordination essentials, and resource management proficiency, nurses will discover newfound efficiency in their workflows. This planner serves not merely as a repository of information, but as a catalyst for transformation, equipping nurses with the tools they need to streamline their patient care processes with precision and compassion.

As nurses embark on their journey towards enhanced care planning and coordination, this planner stands ready to be their steadfast ally, guiding them towards greater efficiency, improved patient outcomes, and ultimately, the fulfillment of their noble calling in the noble

Chapter 1: Foundations of Care Planning

In the intricate tapestry of nursing practice, the foundation upon which exceptional care is built lies in a thorough understanding of the nursing process. From the initial assessment to the final evaluation, each phase plays a vital role in shaping the trajectory of patient care. This chapter delves deep into the core principles of care planning, providing nurses with the necessary framework to navigate the complexities of their role with confidence and competence.

Understanding the Nursing Process: Assessment, Diagnosis, Planning, Implementation, and Evaluation

At the heart of effective care planning lies the nursing process—a systematic framework that guides nurses through the sequential steps of patient care. Beginning with a comprehensive assessment of the patient's needs, strengths, and preferences, nurses gather essential data to inform their clinical judgment. This is followed by the formulation of a nursing diagnosis, wherein nurses identify actual or potential health problems based on their assessment findings. With a clear diagnosis in hand, nurses proceed to the planning phase, where they develop tailored care plans that outline specific interventions and goals aimed at addressing the identified health concerns. Implementation of these interventions marks the next step, as nurses put their plans into action, providing hands-on care and support to their patients. Finally, the evaluation phase allows nurses to assess the effectiveness of their interventions, make necessary adjustments, and ensure that the patient's health needs are met.

Importance of Holistic Care and Patient-Centered Approaches

In the pursuit of excellence in nursing practice, it is essential to recognize the intrinsic value of holistic care and patient-centered approaches. Beyond treating isolated symptoms or ailments, nurses embrace a holistic perspective that considers the interconnectedness of the mind, body, and spirit. By acknowledging the multifaceted nature of human health, nurses can provide comprehensive care that addresses not only physical ailments but also emotional, social, and spiritual needs.

Central to this philosophy is the concept of patient-centered care, which places the patient at the forefront of decision-making and care-planning processes. By actively involving patients in their care, nurses foster a sense of empowerment, autonomy, and trust, laying the groundwork for collaborative partnerships that drive positive health outcomes.

Introduction to the Planner's Structure and Features

As nurses embark on their journey toward mastering the art of care planning, this planner serves as an invaluable resource, guiding them through each phase of the nursing process with clarity and precision. Structured to align seamlessly with the principles of assessment, diagnosis, planning, implementation, and evaluation, this planner offers a comprehensive toolkit equipped with customizable templates, assessment tools, and evidence-based guidelines.

Through its user-friendly interface and intuitive design, nurses can easily navigate the planner's features, ensuring efficient workflow management and seamless integration into their daily practice. From organizing patient assessments to documenting care plans and tracking outcomes, this planner empowers nurses to streamline their care planning processes while upholding the highest standards of quality and patient-centered care.

As nurses immerse themselves in the foundational principles of care planning, they will find in this planner a trusted companion and ally—a beacon of guidance and support on their journey toward excellence in nursing practice.

Chapter 2: Scheduling Mastery

In the fast-paced world of nursing, effective schedule management is essential for maintaining high standards of patient care while ensuring personal well-being and professional satisfaction. This chapter delves into the art of scheduling mastery, offering nurses practical strategies and time management techniques to navigate the demands of their busy schedules with grace and efficiency.

Strategies for Managing Busy Nursing Schedules Effectively

Navigating a busy nursing schedule requires a strategic approach that balances the needs of patients, colleagues, and personal commitments. This section explores various strategies for optimizing schedule management, including the use of scheduling software, delegation of tasks, and effective communication with team members. By leveraging technology and collaborating with colleagues, nurses can streamline their schedules, minimize conflicts, and maximize productivity in their daily workflows.

Utilizing Time Management Techniques to Prioritize Tasks and Appointments

At the core of scheduling mastery lies the ability to prioritize tasks and appointments effectively. This section introduces nurses to proven time management techniques, such as the Eisenhower Matrix, the Pomodoro Technique, and task batching. By categorizing tasks based on urgency and importance, nurses can allocate their time and energy more efficiently, ensuring that critical patient care activities take precedence while still addressing other essential responsibilities.

Tips for Avoiding Burnout and Maintaining Work-Life Balance

As dedicated caregivers, nurses often find themselves balancing demanding work schedules with personal commitments and responsibilities. This section offers practical tips and strategies for nurses to prevent burnout and foster a healthy work-life balance. From setting boundaries and practicing self-care to seeking support from colleagues and supervisors, nurses will discover actionable steps to preserve their well-being and sustain their passion for nursing over the long term.

By mastering the art of scheduling, nurses can not only enhance their efficiency and effectiveness in delivering patient care but also safeguard their own physical and emotional health. As they implement the strategies and techniques outlined in this chapter, nurses will find themselves better equipped to navigate the challenges of their profession with resilience, purpose, and a renewed sense of balance.

Chapter 3: Assessment and Documentation

Thorough and accurate patient assessment, coupled with meticulous documentation, form the cornerstone of nursing practice. This chapter delves into the essential components of assessment and documentation, providing nurses with guidance on conducting comprehensive assessments, adhering to best practices in documentation, and harnessing technology to enhance these critical processes.

Guidance on Thorough and Accurate Patient Assessment

Effective patient assessment is essential for identifying health concerns, establishing baseline data, and formulating individualized care plans. This section offers nurses comprehensive guidance on conducting thorough assessments across various dimensions of patient health, including physical, psychological, social, and environmental factors. By honing their assessment skills and adopting a holistic approach, nurses can gain valuable insights into their patients' needs and tailor their care plans accordingly.

Best Practices for Documenting Patient Information and Care Plans

Accurate and timely documentation is essential for ensuring continuity of care, facilitating communication among healthcare providers, and meeting legal and regulatory requirements. This section outlines best practices for documenting patient information and care plans, emphasizing the importance of clarity, completeness, and confidentiality. From documenting vital signs and medication administration to recording nursing interventions and patient responses, nurses will learn how to maintain meticulous documentation that supports high-quality patient care.

Using Technology to Enhance Assessment and Documentation Processes

In an increasingly digitized healthcare landscape, technology plays a crucial role in streamlining assessment and documentation processes. This section explores the various ways in which nurses can leverage technology to enhance the efficiency and accuracy of their workflows. From electronic health records (EHRs) and mobile health applications to point-of-care documentation tools and telehealth platforms, nurses will discover innovative solutions that enable seamless data capture, analysis, and sharing across healthcare settings. By mastering the art of assessment and documentation and harnessing the power of technology, nurses can elevate the quality of care they provide, improve patient outcomes, and enhance their professional practice. As they integrate the principles and strategies outlined in this chapter into their daily routines, nurses will emerge as confident and competent caregivers, equipped to meet the evolving needs of their patients and healthcare organizations alike.

Chapter 4: Care Coordination Essentials

Effective care coordination lies at the heart of delivering high-quality, patient-centered healthcare. This chapter explores the essential components of care coordination, offering nurses valuable insights and practical strategies for collaborating with interdisciplinary teams, communicating effectively with patients and families, and navigating the complex landscape of healthcare systems and referrals.

Techniques for Collaborating with Interdisciplinary Teams

In today's healthcare environment, patient care often involves collaboration among diverse healthcare professionals, each bringing their unique expertise to the table. This section provides nurses with techniques for fostering effective collaboration within interdisciplinary teams, including clear communication, active listening, and mutual respect. By embracing a collaborative approach to care, nurses can harness the collective strengths of the team to optimize patient outcomes and promote continuity of care.

Effective Communication Strategies with Patients, Families, and Colleagues

Communication lies at the heart of effective care coordination, serving as the linchpin that connects patients, families, and healthcare providers. This section explores communication strategies that enable nurses to build rapport, establish trust, and ensure clarity in their interactions with patients, families, and colleagues. From empathetic listening and open-ended questioning to assertive communication and conflict resolution techniques, nurses will learn how to navigate challenging conversations with confidence and compassion.

Resources for Navigating Complex Healthcare Systems and Referrals

Navigating the complex landscape of healthcare systems, resources, and referrals can be daunting for both patients and healthcare providers alike. This section equips nurses with the knowledge and resources they need to navigate these complexities effectively. From understanding insurance coverage and accessing community resources to facilitating seamless transitions of care and coordinating specialty referrals, nurses will discover practical strategies for guiding patients through the healthcare maze with ease and efficiency.

By mastering the essentials of care coordination, nurses can play a central role in ensuring that patients receive the right care, at the right time, and in the right setting. As they implement the techniques and strategies outlined in this chapter, nurses will emerge as skilled facilitators of care, capable of navigating complex healthcare systems, fostering collaboration among interdisciplinary teams, and empowering patients to achieve optimal health outcomes.

Chapter 5: Resource Management

Effective resource management is essential for nurses to optimize patient care outcomes while navigating the constraints of healthcare budgets and resources. This chapter delves into the principles of resource management, offering nurses practical strategies for maximizing resources, budgeting efficiently, and incorporating evidence-based practices into care planning.

Maximizing Resources to Optimize Patient Care Outcomes

Nurses are entrusted with the responsibility of delivering high-quality care while maximizing the use of available resources. This section explores strategies for optimizing resource utilization, including efficient staffing models, judicious use of supplies and equipment, and leveraging technology to streamline workflows. By maximizing resources without compromising quality, nurses can ensure that patients receive the care they need in a timely and cost-effective manner.

Budgeting Tips for Managing Healthcare Resources Efficiently

In today's healthcare landscape, financial considerations play a significant role in decision-making at all levels of care delivery. This section provides nurses with practical budgeting tips and strategies for managing healthcare resources efficiently. From tracking expenses and identifying cost-saving opportunities to advocating for resource allocation that prioritizes patient care, nurses will learn how to navigate budget constraints while maintaining high standards of care.

Incorporating Evidence-Based Practices and Guidelines into Care Planning

Evidence-based practice serves as a guiding principle for nurses seeking to deliver the most effective and efficient care to their patients. This section explores the importance of incorporating evidence-based practices and clinical guidelines into care planning processes. By staying abreast of the latest research findings and best practices in nursing, nurses can ensure that their care plans are grounded in sound evidence, leading to improved patient outcomes and satisfaction. By mastering the principles of resource management and incorporating evidence-based practices into their care planning processes, nurses can make a significant impact on patient care outcomes while maximizing the use of available resources. As they implement the strategies outlined in this chapter, nurses will emerge as effective stewards of healthcare resources, capable of delivering high-quality care that is both efficient and cost-effective.

Chapter 6: Self-Care and Professional Development

In the demanding and often emotionally taxing field of nursing, prioritizing self-care and ongoing professional development is essential for maintaining physical, emotional, and mental well-being. This chapter explores the importance of self-care, strategies for managing stress and preventing compassion fatigue, and opportunities for continuous professional growth and development.

Importance of Self-Care for Nurses' Physical, Emotional, and Mental Well-being

Nurses are dedicated caregivers, often placing the needs of others above their own. However, neglecting self-care can lead to physical exhaustion, emotional burnout, and diminished mental well-being. This section highlights the importance of prioritizing self-care as a foundational aspect of nursing practice. From maintaining a healthy work-life balance and engaging in regular exercise to practicing mindfulness and seeking social support, nurses will discover strategies for nurturing their physical, emotional, and mental health amidst the demands of their profession.

Strategies for Managing Stress and Preventing Compassion Fatigue

Nursing is inherently stressful, with nurses routinely facing challenging situations, complex patient care needs, and emotionally demanding experiences. This section provides nurses with practical strategies for managing stress and preventing compassion fatigue. From adopting stress-relief techniques such as deep breathing exercises and mindfulness meditation to establishing healthy boundaries and seeking peer support, nurses will learn how to safeguard their well-being and sustain their passion for nursing over the long term.

Opportunities for Professional Growth and Continuing Education

Nursing is a dynamic profession that offers endless opportunities for growth and development. This section explores the various avenues for nurses to pursue professional growth and continuing education. From attending conferences and workshops to pursuing advanced degrees and specialty certifications, nurses will discover a wealth of opportunities to expand their knowledge, enhance their skills, and advance their careers. By investing in lifelong learning and professional development, nurses can stay abreast of the latest advancements in nursing practice and position themselves as leaders in their fields.

By prioritizing self-care, managing stress effectively, and embracing opportunities for professional growth and development, nurses can cultivate resilience, enhance their well-being, and thrive in their nursing careers. As they implement the strategies outlined in this chapter, nurses will emerge as empowered caregivers, equipped to provide compassionate and high-quality care to their patients while nurturing their own health and professional fulfillment.

Chapter 7: Ethical Considerations in Care Planning

Navigating ethical dilemmas is an inherent aspect of nursing practice, particularly in the realm of care planning and coordination. This chapter delves into the complex ethical considerations that nurses may encounter, offering strategies for addressing these issues while upholding patient autonomy, dignity, and well-being. Through the exploration of case studies, nurses will gain insights into ethical decision-making processes and learn how to navigate challenging situations with integrity and compassion.

Discussion on Ethical Dilemmas Nurses May Encounter in Care Planning and Coordination Care planning and coordination often present nurses with ethical dilemmas that require careful consideration and ethical reflection. This section explores common ethical dilemmas encountered in nursing practice, such as balancing the principle of beneficence with respect for patient autonomy, navigating conflicts of interest, and managing competing priorities in care delivery. By engaging in thoughtful discussion and reflection, nurses will develop a deeper understanding of the ethical complexities inherent in their role as caregivers.

Strategies for Addressing Ethical Issues While Upholding Patient Autonomy and Dignity

Ethical decision-making in nursing requires a commitment to upholding the principles of autonomy, beneficence, nonmaleficence, and justice. This section offers nurses practical strategies for addressing ethical issues while safeguarding patient autonomy and dignity. From engaging in open and honest communication with patients and families to advocating for patients' rights and preferences, nurses will learn how to navigate ethical dilemmas with sensitivity, empathy, and respect for individual values and beliefs.

Case Studies Illustrating Ethical Decision-Making in Nursing Practice

Real-life case studies provide valuable opportunities for nurses to apply ethical principles to complex clinical scenarios. This section presents a series of case studies illustrating ethical dilemmas commonly encountered in care planning and coordination. Through guided analysis and discussion, nurses will explore the various factors at play in each scenario, consider the implications of different courses of action, and develop critical thinking skills that enable them to make ethically sound decisions in their practice.

By engaging with the ethical considerations inherent in care planning and coordination, nurses can strengthen their ethical reasoning skills, enhance their ability to navigate challenging situations and uphold the highest standards of integrity and professionalism in their practice. As they grapple with ethical dilemmas and explore strategies for ethical decision-making, nurses will emerge as ethical leaders, dedicated to promoting the well-being and dignity of their patients above all else.

Chapter 8: Cultural Competence and Diversity in Patient Care

Cultural competence and diversity are integral components of providing holistic, patient-centered care. This chapter explores the importance of cultural competence in nursing practice, offering practical tips for navigating cultural differences and language barriers in care planning, and promoting diversity and inclusion in healthcare settings.

Importance of Cultural Competence in Providing Holistic and Respectful Care

Cultural competence is the ability to effectively interact with individuals from diverse cultural backgrounds, acknowledging and respecting their beliefs, values, and practices. This section underscores the significance of cultural competence in nursing practice, emphasizing its role in fostering trust, enhancing communication, and promoting positive health outcomes. By recognizing and honoring cultural differences, nurses can provide more holistic and respectful care that meets the unique needs of each patient.

Tips for Navigating Cultural Differences and Language Barriers in Care Planning

Cultural differences and language barriers can pose challenges in care planning and coordination, impacting the quality and effectiveness of patient care. This section offers practical tips for nurses to navigate these challenges effectively. From engaging in cross-cultural communication and using interpreters or language assistance services to conducting cultural assessments and incorporating culturally sensitive interventions into care plans, nurses will learn how to bridge cultural divides and provide culturally competent care to diverse patient populations.

Promoting Diversity and Inclusion in Healthcare Settings

Promoting diversity and inclusion in healthcare settings is essential for creating environments that are welcoming, respectful, and equitable for all patients and healthcare providers. This section explores strategies for promoting diversity and inclusion in nursing practice, including fostering cultural awareness and sensitivity among healthcare teams, advocating for policies and practices that promote equity and access to care, and actively engaging with diverse communities to understand their unique needs and preferences.

By embracing cultural competence and diversity in patient care, nurses can enhance the quality of care they provide, strengthen patient-provider relationships, and contribute to more equitable and inclusive healthcare systems. As they implement the strategies outlined in this chapter, nurses will emerge as advocates for cultural humility and champions for diversity and inclusion in nursing practice and beyond.

Chapter 9: Technology Integration for Enhanced Care Coordination

In the rapidly evolving landscape of healthcare, technology plays a pivotal role in enhancing care coordination, improving communication among healthcare providers, and optimizing patient outcomes. This chapter provides an overview of digital tools and software designed to streamline care coordination, offers tips for selecting and implementing technology solutions that meet nurses' needs and addresses ethical considerations and privacy concerns related to electronic health records (EHRs) and telehealth.

Overview of Digital Tools and Software Designed to Streamline Care Coordination

A multitude of digital tools and software solutions are available to facilitate care coordination and communication among healthcare providers. This section provides an overview of these tools, including EHR systems, secure messaging platforms, care coordination applications, and telehealth platforms. By harnessing the power of technology, nurses can streamline communication, share critical patient information in real time, and collaborate more effectively with interdisciplinary teams to deliver seamless and coordinated care.

Tips for Selecting and Implementing Technology Solutions That Meet Nurses' Needs

Selecting and implementing technology solutions requires careful consideration of nurses' needs, preferences, and workflows. This section offers practical tips for nurses to navigate the process of selecting and implementing technology solutions effectively. From conducting needs assessments and evaluating different software options to providing comprehensive training and ongoing staff support, nurses will learn how to ensure the successful adoption and integration of technology into their care coordination processes.

Ethical Considerations and Privacy Concerns Related to Electronic Health Records and Telehealth

While technology offers numerous benefits for care coordination, it also raises ethical considerations and privacy concerns that must be addressed. This section explores the ethical implications of using EHRs and telehealth platforms, including issues related to patient confidentiality, data security, and informed consent. Nurses will learn how to navigate these ethical challenges responsibly, ensuring that patient privacy is protected and ethical principles are upheld in the use of technology for care coordination.

By integrating technology into care coordination processes thoughtfully and responsibly, nurses can enhance communication, collaboration, and efficiency in delivering patient care. As they navigate the complexities of selecting, implementing, and using technology solutions, nurses will emerge as adept users of technology, equipped to leverage its full potential to improve patient outcomes and enhance the quality of care they provide.

Chapter 10: Emergency Preparedness and Crisis Management

In healthcare, emergencies and crises can arise unexpectedly, requiring nurses to respond swiftly and effectively to ensure the safety and well-being of patients and staff. This chapter explores strategies for developing emergency response plans and protocols, outlines the role of nurses in disaster preparedness and mitigation efforts, and presents case studies highlighting effective crisis management in healthcare settings.

Strategies for Developing Emergency Response Plans and Protocols

Developing comprehensive emergency response plans and protocols is essential for healthcare organizations to effectively manage emergencies and crises. This section provides nurses with strategies for developing robust plans that address a range of potential scenarios, including natural disasters, infectious disease outbreaks, and mass casualty incidents. By establishing clear communication channels, defining roles and responsibilities, and conducting regular drills and simulations, nurses can ensure that their organizations are well-prepared to respond to emergencies effectively and minimize disruptions to patient care.

Role of Nurses in Disaster Preparedness and Mitigation Efforts

Nurses play a critical role in disaster preparedness and mitigation efforts, serving as frontline responders and leaders in times of crisis. This section outlines the various roles and responsibilities that nurses may assume during emergencies, including triage, patient care, resource management, and communication coordination. By leveraging their clinical expertise, leadership skills, and knowledge of community resources, nurses can make significant contributions to disaster preparedness and mitigation efforts, helping to safeguard the health and safety of their patients and communities.

Case Studies Highlighting Effective Crisis Management in Healthcare Settings

Real-life case studies provide valuable insights into effective crisis management strategies and highlight the importance of preparedness, coordination, and adaptability in responding to emergencies. This section presents a series of case studies that illustrate successful crisis management efforts in healthcare settings, including responses to natural disasters, infectious disease outbreaks, and other emergencies. By analyzing these case studies, nurses can gain valuable lessons learned and best practices that can inform their emergency preparedness efforts and enhance their ability to respond effectively to future crises.

By embracing a proactive approach to emergency preparedness and crisis management, nurses can play a pivotal role in safeguarding the health and safety of their patients, colleagues, and communities. As they develop and implement emergency response plans, assume leadership roles in disaster preparedness efforts, and learn from real-life case studies, nurses will emerge as resilient and resourceful responders, capable of effectively managing emergencies and ensuring continuity of care in the face of adversity.

Chapter 11: Quality Improvement and Patient Safety

Quality improvement and patient safety are paramount in ensuring the delivery of safe, effective, and patient-centered care. This chapter explores the importance of quality improvement initiatives in enhancing patient outcomes, techniques for monitoring and evaluating the effectiveness of care plans, and strategies for implementing evidence-based practices to improve patient safety and satisfaction.

Importance of Quality Improvement Initiatives in Enhancing Patient Outcomes

Quality improvement initiatives are essential for identifying areas for improvement, implementing changes, and evaluating the impact of these changes on patient outcomes. This section underscores the importance of continuous quality improvement in nursing practice, emphasizing its role in enhancing patient safety, reducing medical errors, and improving clinical outcomes. By embracing a culture of quality improvement, nurses can drive positive change, foster innovation, and deliver care that meets the highest standards of excellence.

Techniques for Monitoring and Evaluating the Effectiveness of Care Plans

Monitoring and evaluating the effectiveness of care plans are essential components of quality improvement efforts. This section offers nurses practical techniques for assessing the impact of care interventions on patient outcomes, including the use of performance metrics, outcome measures, and quality indicators. By collecting and analyzing data systematically, nurses can identify areas for improvement, track progress over time, and make informed decisions to optimize patient care delivery.

Implementing Evidence-Based Practices to Improve Patient Safety and Satisfaction

Evidence-based practices serve as the foundation for delivering high-quality, safe, and effective patient care. This section explores strategies for implementing evidence-based practices to improve patient safety and satisfaction. From conducting literature reviews and critically appraising research evidence to incorporating best practices into care plans and workflows, nurses will learn how to integrate evidence-based care principles into their daily practice. By aligning care delivery with the best available evidence, nurses can enhance patient outcomes, reduce variability in practice, and promote a culture of excellence in patient care. By embracing quality improvement initiatives, monitoring and evaluating care effectiveness, and implementing evidence-based practices, nurses can drive continuous improvement in patient care delivery. As they engage with the strategies outlined in this chapter, nurses will emerge as champions for quality and safety, committed to delivering care that is safe, effective, and patient-centered.

Chapter 12: Leadership and Advocacy in Nursing

Leadership and advocacy are integral aspects of nursing practice, empowering nurses to drive positive change, influence policy decisions, and champion the well-being of patients and communities. This chapter explores opportunities for nurses to take on leadership roles in care planning and coordination, advocacy strategies for promoting policy changes and improving healthcare systems, and inspiring stories of nurse leaders making a difference in their communities.

Opportunities for Nurses to Take on Leadership Roles in Care Planning and Coordination

Nurses possess unique clinical expertise, critical thinking skills, and interpersonal abilities that make them well-suited for leadership roles in care planning and coordination. This section highlights the various opportunities for nurses to assume leadership positions within healthcare organizations, interdisciplinary teams, and community settings. From serving as charge nurses and nurse managers to leading quality improvement initiatives and serving on committees, nurses can leverage their leadership skills to drive innovation, improve care delivery, and enhance patient outcomes.

Advocacy Strategies for Promoting Policy Changes and Improving Healthcare Systems
Advocacy is a powerful tool for nurses to influence policy decisions, address systemic issues, and advocate for the needs of patients and communities. This section explores advocacy strategies that nurses can employ to promote policy changes and improve healthcare systems at local, regional, and national levels. From grassroots organizing and coalition-building to engaging with policymakers and advocating for evidence-based policies, nurses will learn how to effectively advocate for changes that advance the interests of patients, promote health equity, and strengthen the nursing profession.

Inspiring Stories of Nurse Leaders Making a Difference in Their Communities
Real-life stories of nurse leaders serve as inspiration and motivation for nurses seeking to

make a difference in their communities. This section presents a series of inspiring stories highlighting the transformative impact of nurse leaders in diverse settings and contexts. From leading initiatives to address health disparities and improve access to care to advocating for changes in healthcare policy and shaping the future of nursing education, these stories showcase the leadership potential of nurses and the profound difference they can make in the lives of individuals and communities.

By embracing leadership roles and advocacy opportunities, nurses can harness their collective voice and influence to drive positive change in healthcare. As they engage with the strategies and stories presented in this chapter, nurses will be inspired to lead with courage, compassion, and commitment, leaving a lasting legacy of impact and innovation in their communities and beyond.

Chapter 13: Innovations in Nursing Practice

Innovation lies at the heart of nursing practice, driving forward-thinking approaches to care planning, coordination, and delivery. This chapter explores innovative approaches to care planning and coordination, showcases examples of nurse-led initiatives and projects driving positive change in healthcare, and offers tips for embracing creativity and new ideas in nursing practice.

Exploration of Innovative Approaches to Care Planning and Coordination

Innovation in care planning and coordination involves exploring new ideas, technologies, and methodologies to enhance patient care outcomes and streamline workflows. This section delves into innovative approaches that nurses can adopt to optimize care delivery, such as the integration of artificial intelligence and machine learning into clinical decision-making, the implementation of telehealth and remote monitoring solutions, and the development of patient-centered care models that prioritize collaboration and shared decision-making. By embracing innovation, nurses can stay at the forefront of advancements in healthcare and drive continuous improvement in patient care.

Examples of Nurse-Led Initiatives and Projects Driving Positive Change in Healthcare

Nurses are innovators and change agents, leading initiatives and projects that transform the landscape of healthcare. This section showcases examples of nurse-led initiatives that have made a significant impact on patient outcomes, healthcare delivery, and system improvement. From developing innovative care delivery models to implementing quality improvement projects and spearheading community health initiatives, these examples highlight the diverse ways in which nurses are driving positive change and shaping the future of healthcare.

Tips for Embracing Creativity and Embracing New Ideas in Nursing Practice

Embracing creativity and new ideas is essential for fostering innovation and driving positive change in nursing practice. This section offers practical tips for nurses to cultivate a culture of creativity and innovation in their practice settings. From fostering a supportive and collaborative work environment to seeking out opportunities for professional development and networking, nurses will learn how to nurture their creative instincts, challenge the status quo, and embrace new ideas that have the potential to revolutionize patient care delivery.

By embracing innovation, nurses can drive positive change, improve patient outcomes, and shape the future of healthcare. As they engage with the innovative approaches, nurse-led initiatives, and creativity tips presented in this chapter, nurses will be inspired to think outside the box, push boundaries, and lead with innovation in their practice settings.

Chapter 14: Future Trends and Challenges in Nursing

The future of nursing practice is marked by dynamic trends and evolving challenges that shape the landscape of healthcare delivery. This chapter engages in a discussion on emerging trends and challenges, explores opportunities for nurses to adapt and thrive in an evolving healthcare landscape, and provides recommendations for staying informed and prepared for future developments.

Discussion on Emerging Trends and Challenges Shaping the Future of Nursing Practice

The healthcare landscape is constantly evolving, driven by advances in technology, changes in demographics, and shifts in healthcare policy and practice. This section delves into emerging trends and challenges that are shaping the future of nursing practice. Topics may include the integration of artificial intelligence and robotics into healthcare delivery, the rise of telehealth and virtual care models, the impact of population aging on healthcare demands, and the evolving role of nurses in addressing social determinants of health. By understanding these trends and challenges, nurses can anticipate future developments and proactively prepare for the changing healthcare landscape.

Opportunities for Nurses to Adapt and Thrive in an Evolving Healthcare Landscape

Despite the challenges posed by a rapidly changing healthcare environment, there are numerous opportunities for nurses to adapt and thrive. This section explores the various ways in which nurses can leverage their skills, expertise, and leadership to navigate the complexities of the future healthcare landscape. Opportunities may include pursuing advanced education and training, specializing in emerging areas of practice, advocating for policy changes that support nursing practice, and embracing interdisciplinary collaboration to address complex healthcare needs. By seizing these opportunities, nurses can position themselves as key drivers of innovation and change in healthcare.

Recommendations for Staying Informed and Prepared for Future Developments
Staying informed and prepared for future developments is essential for nurses to remain effective and relevant in their practice. This section provides recommendations for nurses to stay abreast of emerging trends, research findings, and policy changes that impact nursing practice. Recommendations may include participating in professional development activities, joining professional organizations and networks, engaging in lifelong learning, and seeking out mentorship and leadership opportunities. By staying informed and proactive, nurses can adapt to the evolving healthcare landscape and continue to deliver high-quality care that meets the needs of patients and communities.

As nurses navigate the future of nursing practice, they must remain adaptable, innovative, and forward-thinking. By engaging with the trends, challenges, and opportunities presented in this chapter, nurses can position themselves as leaders and change agents in shaping the future of healthcare delivery. Through ongoing learning, collaboration, and advocacy, nurses can ensure that they are well-equipped to meet the evolving needs of patients and communities in the years to come.

Chapter 15: Reflection and Goal Setting

Reflection and goal setting are essential components of professional growth and development for nurses. This chapter encourages nurses to reflect on their practice and personal growth, provides tools and exercises for setting short-term and long-term goals in care planning and coordination, and offers strategies for celebrating achievements and maintaining motivation in nursing practice.

Encouragement for Nurses to Reflect on Their Practice and Personal Growth

Reflection allows nurses to pause, examine their experiences, and gain insights that can inform their practice and personal growth. This section encourages nurses to engage in reflective practice, whether through journaling, peer discussions, or structured reflection exercises. By reflecting on their experiences, challenges, and successes, nurses can gain valuable insights, identify areas for improvement, and enhance their professional competence and resilience.

Tools and Exercises for Setting Short-Term and Long-Term Goals in Care Planning and Coordination

Goal setting is a powerful tool for nurses to translate their reflections into actionable plans for personal and professional development. This section provides nurses with tools and exercises for setting SMART (Specific, Measurable, Achievable, Relevant, Time-bound) goals in care planning and coordination. Nurses will learn how to identify areas for improvement, set realistic and achievable goals, and develop action plans that outline steps for achieving their objectives. By setting clear goals, nurses can stay focused, motivated, and accountable as they work towards continuous improvement in their practice.

Strategies for Celebrating Achievements and Maintaining Motivation in Nursing Practice

Celebrating achievements is essential for recognizing progress, boosting morale, and sustaining motivation in nursing practice. This section offers strategies for nurses to celebrate their successes, whether big or small. From acknowledging milestones and accomplishments in team meetings to rewarding oneself for achieving personal goals, nurses will learn how to cultivate a culture of celebration and positivity in their practice settings. By celebrating achievements, nurses can reinforce their commitment to excellence and maintain a sense of fulfillment and satisfaction in their work.

By engaging in reflection, setting goals, and celebrating achievements, nurses can cultivate a culture of continuous learning and improvement in their practice. As they implement the tools, exercises, and strategies outlined in this chapter, nurses will develop the skills, resilience, and motivation needed to thrive in their nursing careers and make a positive impact on patient care and outcomes.

Conclusion

As we conclude this planner, it's important to reflect on the key concepts and tools provided to support nurses in their practice of care, compassion, and coordination. Throughout this planner, we have explored essential topics such as care planning, scheduling mastery, assessment and documentation, and ethical considerations, among others.

Recap of Key Concepts and Tools Provided in the Planner

We have provided nurses with practical strategies, techniques, and resources to enhance their practice and improve patient outcomes. From developing comprehensive care plans to leveraging technology for streamlined coordination, nurses have access to a wealth of tools and information to support their professional growth and development.

Encouragement for Nurses to Prioritize Care, Compassion, and Coordination in Their Practice

As nurses, your dedication to providing high-quality care, showing compassion, and facilitating effective coordination is at the heart of what you do every day. In the face of challenges and demands, it's essential to prioritize these core values and principles in your practice. By embracing care, compassion, and coordination, you can make a meaningful difference in the lives of your patients and contribute to a culture of excellence in healthcare.

Invitation to Share Feedback and Success Stories Using the Planner

We value your feedback and encourage you to share your experiences, challenges, and success stories as you implement the strategies and tools provided in this planner. Your feedback helps us continuously improve and refine our resources to better meet the needs of nurses like you. Additionally, sharing your success stories inspires and motivates others in the nursing community, fostering a sense of collaboration and support.

In closing, we extend our sincere appreciation to all nurses for their unwavering dedication, compassion, and commitment to excellence in patient care. As you continue your journey in nursing, remember that you are valued, respected, and appreciated for the vital role you play in promoting health and healing. Thank you for all that you do, and we wish you continued success and fulfillment in your nursing practice.

Appendix: Additional Resources

In this appendix, you will find a collection of valuable resources to further support your practice and ongoing professional development. These resources include templates for care plans, assessment forms, and scheduling tools, as well as recommended readings, websites, and organizations for further learning and support. Templates for Care Plans, Assessment Forms, and Scheduling Tools

1. Care Plan Template: A comprehensive template to guide the development of patient-centered care plans, including sections for assessment data, nursing diagnoses, goals, interventions, and evaluation.
2. Assessment Form: A structured form for conducting thorough and systematic patient assessments, capturing vital signs, health history, medication information, and other relevant data.
3. Scheduling Tool: A customizable tool to help nurses effectively manage their

schedules, prioritize tasks, and coordinate care for multiple patients or clients.
Recommended Readings, Websites, and Organizations for Further Learning and Support

1. Books:
    - "Nursing Care Plans: Diagnoses, Interventions, and Outcomes" by Meg Gulanick and Judith Myers
    - "Evidence-Based Practice in Nursing & Healthcare: A Guide to Best Practice" by Bernadette Melnyk and Ellen Fineout-Overholt
2. Websites:
    - American Nurses Association (ANA): A professional organization offering resources, guidelines, and advocacy initiatives for nurses across all specialties. Website: www.nursingworld.org
    - National Institute of Nursing Research (NINR): A branch of the National Institutes of Health (NIH) focused on advancing nursing science and promoting the health

and well-being of individuals,
families, and communities.
Website: www.ninr.nih.gov

3. Organizations:

   - Sigma Theta Tau International Honor Society of Nursing: An honor society that recognizes excellence in nursing practice, education, and research, providing networking opportunities, educational resources, and leadership development programs. Website: www.sigmanursing.org
   - National League for Nursing (NLN): An organization dedicated to promoting excellence in nursing education and advancing the quality of nursing care, offering professional development resources, accreditation services, and advocacy initiatives. Website: www.nln.org

These resources are designed to complement the content provided in this planner and support

your continued growth and success as a nurse.
Whether you are seeking guidance on care
planning, looking for evidence-based practice
guidelines, or exploring opportunities for
professional networking and development, these
resources offer valuable insights and support to
enhance your practice and improve patient
outcomes.

Index

The index provides a comprehensive reference guide to specific topics, tools, and concepts discussed throughout the book. It serves as a valuable resource for quick and easy navigation, allowing readers to locate information on key subjects and access relevant tools and resources. Entries are organized alphabetically, making it convenient to find relevant information on care planning, assessment forms, scheduling tools, recommended readings, websites, and organizations. The index enhances the usability and accessibility of the book, enabling readers to efficiently locate and reference content as needed.

www.ingramcontent.com/pod-product-compliance
Lightning Source LLC
Chambersburg PA
CBHW070801250726
48662CB00004B/1924